Table of Contents

INTRODUCTION

Cannabis has been used for thousands of years both medically and recreationally by people across the globe. In the United States, cannabis has been federally illegal since the 1930s and was given a Schedule I substance classification in 1970 under the Controlled Substances Act (CSA). In 1996, California became the first state to legalize medical cannabis. Colorado and Washington were the first states to legalize recreational cannabis in 2012.

Since then, many states have passed legislation to create medical cannabis programs and/or allow recreational cannabis consumption for adults 21 and older. Initially, medical cannabis and its potential therapeutic benefits drove legalization efforts along with activists dedicated to reforming racist and destructive drug policies that fuel the U.S. prison industrial complex.

Cannabis remains federally illegal in the U.S. today. However, with the liberalization of cannabis policies across dozens of states, more research has been allowed to be conducted both on the potential medical benefits of using cannabis and for separating fact from fiction when it comes to the downsides of cannabis use.

Since the oldest days, cannabis has been used differently and in abundance — mostly as hemp for manufacturing ropes, textiles, etc. However, it came to prominence throughout the last couple hundred years, with its legality status changing several times in the US only, with the first official restriction being imposed back in 1937.

Today, the US and some other countries are removing restrictions steadily. As a result, stats show that cannabis legalization appears to be creating unseen revenue. Some $12 billion were projected for 2019, with 2017 generating around $10 billion.

Uruguay was the first country to fully legalize cannabis use in 2013, while Canada was the second state to do the same five years later. That year, surveys reported that roughly two-thirds of the US legal-age population supported cannabis legalization, as opposed to only 12% of the population which supported legalization in 1969.

CHAPTER ONE

HISTORY OF CANNABIS

Cannabis sativa is one of the world's oldest cultivated plants (Russo, 2007). Although the earliest written records of the human use of cannabis date from the 6th century B.C. (ca. 2,600 cal BP), existing evidence suggests that its use in Europe and East Asia started in the early Holocene (ca. 8,000 cal BP) (Long et al., 2016). Many 19th-century practitioners ascribed medicinal properties to cannabis after the drug found its way to Europe during a period of colonial expansion into Africa and Asia. For example, William B. O'Shaughnessy, an Irish physician working at the Medical College and Hospital in Calcutta, first introduced cannabis (Indian hemp) to Western medicine as a treatment for tetanus and other convulsive diseases (O'Shaughnessy, 1840). At approximately the same time, French physician Jean-Jacques Moreau de Tours experimented with the use of cannabis preparations for the treatment of mental disorders (Moreau de Tours, 1845). Soon after, in 1851, cannabis was included in the 3rd edition of the Pharmacopoeia of the United States (USP). Subsequent revisions of the USP described in detail how to prepare extracts and tinctures of dried cannabis flowers to be used as analgesic, hypnotic, and anticonvulsant (Russo, 2007; U.S. Pharmacopoeial Convention, 1916). Growing concerns about cannabis resulted in the outlawing of cannabis in several states in the early 1900s and federal prohibition of the drug in 1937 with the passage of the Marihuana Tax Act. In response to these concerns, in 1942 the American Medical Association removed cannabis from the 12th edition of U.S. Pharmacopeia (IOM, 1999).

THE CANNABIS PLANT

Cannabis cultivars are considered as part of one genus, Cannabis, family Cannabaceae, order Urticales (Kuddus et al., 2013). Two accepted genera of Cannabaceae are Cannabis and Humulus (hops). There is, however, an ongoing debate concerning the taxonomic differentiation within the Cannabis genus (Laursen, 2015). On the basis of genetic variations, a multitypic genus with at least two putative species, Cannabis sativa and Cannabis indica, has been proposed by some researchers (Clarke and Merlin, 2015; Hillig, 2005). Other researchers have suggested a unique species Cannabis sativa with the genetic differences explained by variations at both the subspecies and the variety level or at a biotype level of putative taxa (Small, 2015).

Chemical Constituents of Cannabis

To date, more than 104 different cannabinoids[1] have been identified in cannabis (ElSohly and Gul, 2014). Other compounds identified include terpenoids, flavonoids, nitrogenous compounds, and more common plant molecules (American Herbal Pharmacopoeia, 2013). Among these, Δ9-tetrahydrocannabinol (THC) has received the most attention for being responsible for the intoxicated state sought after by recreational cannabis users, owing to its ability to act as a partial agonist2 for type-1 cannabinoid (CB1) receptors. Cannabinoids exist mainly in the plant as their carboxylic precursors (Δ9-tetrahydrocannabinolic acid [THCA] and cannabidiolic acid [CBDA]) and are decarboxylated by light or heat while in storage or when combusted (Grotenhermen, 2003). Δ9-THC is synthesized within the glandular trichomes present in the flowers, leaves, and bracts of the female plant. It shares a common precursor, olivetoic acid, with another quantitatively important constituent of Cannabis sativa, cannabidiol (CBD), which is the most abundant cannabinoid in hemp (see Figure 2-1). For this reason, the genetic profile and relative level of expression of the enzymes responsible for their synthesis (genotype), namely THCA synthase and CBDA synthase, determine the chemical composition of a particular cultivar (chemotype).

FIGURE 2-1

Synthetic pathway of the main cannabinoids, Δ9-THC and CBD, from the common precursor, olivetol.

Cannabis plants typically exhibit one of the three main different chemotypes based on the absolute and relative concentrations of Δ9-THCA and CBDA (see Table 2-1), which makes it possible to distinguish among the Δ9-THC-type, or drug-type; the intermediate-type; and the CBD-type cannabis plants grown for fiber (industrial hemp) or seed oil in which the content of Δ9-THC does not exceed 0.3 percent on a dry-weight basis (Chandra et al., 2013). CBD is pharmacologically active, however, and, therefore, classifying cannabis in terms of drug- and fiber-producing seems inaccurate. Both THC- and CBD-types are considered drug-types, and both cultivars could theoretically be exploited to produce fiber.

In a series of studies conducted in the late 1930s and early 1940s, Roger Adams and coworkers isolated cannabinol and CBD from hemp oil and then isomerized CBD into a mixture of two tetrahydrocannabinols with "marihuana-like" physiological activity in dogs, proving their structure except for the final placement of one double bond (Adams et al., 1940a,b). Two years later, tetrahydrocannabinol was first isolated from cannabis resin (Wollner et al., 1942). In 1964, thanks to the development of such potent analytical techniques as nuclear magnetic resonance imaging, Gaoni and Mechoulam were able to identify the position of this elusive double bond, thus resolving the final structure of Δ9-THC (Gaoni and Mechoulam, 1964).

In the late 1980s William Devane and Allyn Howlett first postulated the existence of cannabinoid receptors by showing how synthetic molecules designed to mimic the actions of Δ9-THC were able to bind a selective site in brain membranes, thus inhibiting the intracellular synthesis of cyclic adenosine monophosphate (cAMP) through a G protein–mediated mechanism (Devane et al., 1988). The mapping of cannabinoid-binding sites in the rat brain (Herkenham et al., 1990) and the molecular cloning of the first cannabinoid receptor gene (Matsuda et al.,

1990) subsequently corroborated this hypothesis. Three years later, a second G protein–coupled cannabinoid receptor was cloned from a promyelocytic cell line and termed CB2 (Munro et al., 1993).

Both CB1 and CB2 signal through the transducing G proteins, Gi and Go, and their activation by Δ9-THC or other agonists causes the inhibition of adenylyl cyclase activity, the closing of voltage-gated calcium channels, the opening of inwardly rectifying potassium channels, and the stimulation of mitogen-activated protein kinases such as extracellular signal–regulated kinases (ERKs) and focal adhesion kinases (FAKs) (Mackie, 2006).

The expression pattern of CB1 receptors in brain structures correlates with the psychoactive effects of cannabis. In mammals, high concentrations of CB1 are found in areas that regulate appetite, memory, fear extinction, motor responses, and posture such as the hippocampus, basal ganglia, basolateral amygdala, hypothalamus, and cerebellum (Mackie, 2006). CB1 is also found in a number of nonneural tissues, including the gastrointestinal tract, adipocytes, liver, and skeletal muscle. In addition to CB1, the brain also contains a small number of CB2 receptors, although this subtype is mainly expressed in macrophages and macrophage-derived cells such as microglia, osteoclasts, and osteoblasts (Mackie, 2006).

Pharmacological Properties of Cannabidiol

Cannabidiol was first isolated from hemp oil in 1940 (Adams et al., 1940a) and its structure predicted by chemical methods (Adams et al., 1940b); its fine structure was determined in later studies (Mechoulam and Shvo, 1963). CBD lacks the cannabis-like intoxicating properties of Δ9-THC and, for this reason, has been traditionally considered non-psychoactive. CBD displays very low affinity for CB1 and CB2 cannabinoid receptors (Thomas et al., 2007), but it might be able to negatively modulate CB1 via an allosteric mechanism (Laprairie et al., 2015)3; however, CBD can interfere with the deactivation of the endocannabinoid molecule anandamide, by targeting either its uptake or its enzymatic degradation, catalyzed by fatty-acid amide hydrolase (FAAH), which could indirectly activate CB1 (De Petrocellis et al., 2011; Elmes et al., 2015) (see Box 2-1).

CBD is also a known agonist of serotonin 5-HT1A receptors (Russo et al., 2005) and transient receptor potential vanilloid type 1 (TRPV1) receptors (Bisogno et al., 2001). It can also enhance adenosine receptor signaling by inhibiting adenosine inactivation, suggesting a potential therapeutic role in pain and inflammation (Carrier et al., 2006). The antioxidant and anti-inflammatory properties of this compound may explain its potential neuroprotective actions (Scuderi et al., 2009). Irrespective of the mechanism of action, there is evidence that CBD could potentially be exploited in the treatment and symptom relief of various neurological disorders such as epilepsy and seizures (Hofmann and Frazier, 2013; Jones et al., 2010), psychosis (Leweke et al., 2016), anxiety (Bergamaschi et al., 2011), movement disorders (e.g., Huntington's disease and amyotrophic lateral sclerosis) (de Lago and Fernandez-Ruiz, 2007; Iuvone et al., 2009), and multiple sclerosis (Lakhan and Rowland, 2009).

CANNABIS-DERIVED PRODUCTS

In the United States, cannabis-derived products are consumed for both medical and recreational purposes in a variety of ways. These include smoking or inhaling from cigarettes (joints), pipes (bowls), water pipes (bongs, hookahs), and blunts (cigars filled with cannabis); eating or drinking food products and beverages; or vaporizing the product. These different modes are used to consume different cannabis products, including cannabis "buds" (dried cannabis flowers); cannabis resin (hashish, bubble hash); and cannabis oil (butane honey oil, shatter, wax, crumble). The oil, which may contain up to 75 percent Δ9-THC—versus 5 to 20 percent in the herb or resin (Raber et al., 2015)—is extracted from plant material using organic solvents, such as ethanol, hexane, butane, or supercritical (or subcritical) CO_2, and can be either smoked or vaporized by pressing the extracted oil against the heated surface of an oil rig pipe (dabbing). Cannabinoids can also be absorbed through the skin and mucosal tissues, so topical creams, patches, vaginal sprays, and rectal suppositories are sometimes employed and used as a form of administering Δ9-THC (Brenneisen et al., 1996). A broad selection of cannabis-derived products are also available in the form of food and snack items, beverages, clothing, and health and beauty aid products.

Potency of Cannabis

In the 1990s and early 2000s, the bulk of cannabis consumed in the United States was grown abroad and illicitly imported. The past decade has seen an influx of high-potency cannabis produced within the United States—for example, "sinsemilla"—which is grown from clones rather than from seeds. Data from the U.S. Drug Enforcement Administration (DEA) seizures record a substantial increase in average potency, from 4 percent in 1995 to roughly 12 percent in 2014, both because high-quality U.S.-grown cannabis has taken market share from Mexican imports and because cannabis from both sources has grown in potency (ElSohly et al., 2016; Kilmer, 2014).

Route of Administration

The route of administration of cannabis can affect the onset, intensity, and duration of the psychotropic effects, the effects on organ systems, and the addictive potential and negative consequences associated with its use (Ehrler et al., 2015). The consumption of cannabis causes a particular combination of relaxation and euphoria, commonly referred to as a "high." When cannabis is smoked, Δ9-THC quickly diffuses to the brain, eliciting a perceived high within seconds to minutes. Blood levels of Δ9-THC reach a maximum after about 30 minutes and then rapidly subside within 1 to 3.5 hours (Fabritius et al., 2013;

Huestis et al., 1992). Vaping has an onset, peak, and duration that are similar to those of smoking and produces a similar high (Abrams et al., 2007). "Dabbing," a term for flash-vaporizing butane hash oil-based concentrates, has been reported to offer a different and stronger intoxicating effect than smoking/vaping (Loflin and Earleywine, 2014). By contrast, eating does not produce effects for 30 minutes to 2 hours, and the perceived high is relatively prolonged, lasting 5 to 8 hours or even longer. The slow action of orally ingested cannabis is due to Δ9-THC being absorbed by the intestine and transported to the liver (hepatic first pass) where it is converted into 11-OH-THC, an equipotent and longer-lasting metabolite (Huestis et al., 1992). Edibles make it harder to titrate the intoxicating effects due to the delayed and variable onset. Consequently, edibles have been tied to the ingestion of excessive amounts of cannabis under the misperception that the initial dose had not produced the desired effect (Ghosh and Basu, 2015; MacCoun and Mello, 2015). The availability of edibles has also been associated with increased rates of accidental pediatric ingestion of cannabis (Wang et al., 2014).

Trends in Routes of Administration

There are no high-quality nationally representative data on the prevalence of the non-herbal forms of cannabis (e.g., edibles, oils, and other concentrates), but evidence suggests that they are more commonly used by medical cannabis patients in states with recreational or lenient medical cannabis policies (Daniulaityte et al., 2015; Pacula et al., 2016). Forty percent of 12th-grade past-year users reported using cannabis in edible form in medical cannabis states, versus 26 percent in states without medical cannabis laws (NIDA, 2014). In Washington State, an online survey from 2013 found that, among daily and near-daily cannabis users, 27.5 percent had used edibles, 22.8 percent had used hash resin, and 20.4 percent had "dabbed" in the past week (Kilmer et al., 2013).

Data from recreational cannabis sales in Washington and Colorado provide a glimpse of trends that are specific to markets that have legalized cannabis. In Washington State, herbal cannabis remains dominant, having accounted for two-thirds of all sales revenues in June 2016, but it is losing market share as "cannabis extracts for inhalation" become more popular, at 21 percent in June 2016 as compared with 12 percent 1 year prior. The sales of liquid and solid edibles (9 percent) combined account for most of the remaining sales.4 Non-herbal varieties are even more popular on Colorado's recreational market, where herbal cannabis accounts for a narrow majority (56 percent) and sales of solid concentrates (24 percent) and edibles (13 percent) are on the rise (Castle, 2016).

Partly to provide a guide for the responsible use of non-herbal varieties of cannabis, states that have legalized the recreational cannabis have defined a standard "dose" of THC. Washington State and Colorado have set the standard "dose" of THC as 10 mg, while Oregon chose a lower limit of 5 mg. For perspective, the typical joint size in the United States is 0.66 g (Mariani et al., 2011) and the average potency is 8 percent THC (Fabritius et al., 2013), resulting in an average dose of 8.25 mg THC per joint; higher THC levels ranging from 15–20 percent or higher would yield a THC dose between 9.9–13.2 mg. Occasional users report feeling "high" after consuming only 2–3 mg of THC (Hall and Pacula, 2010); however, users who have developed tolerance to the effects of THC via frequent use may prefer much larger quantities.

CLINICAL FEATURES OF CANNABIS INTOXICATION

During acute cannabis intoxication, the user's sociability and sensitivity to certain stimuli (e.g., colors, music) may be enhanced, the perception of time is altered, and the appetite for sweet and fatty foods is heightened. Some users report feeling relaxed or experiencing a pleasurable "rush" or "buzz" after smoking cannabis (Agrawal et al., 2014). These subjective effects are often associated with decreased short-term memory, dry mouth, and impaired perception and motor skills. When very high blood levels of Δ9-THC are attained, the person may experience panic attacks, paranoid thoughts, and hallucinations (Li et al., 2014). Furthermore, as legalized medical and recreational cannabis availability increase nationwide, the impairment of driving abilities during acute intoxication has become a public safety issue.

In addition to Δ9-THC dosage, two main factors influence the intensity and duration of acute intoxication: individual differences in the rate of absorption and metabolism of Δ9-THC, and the loss of sensitivity to its pharmacological actions. Prolonged CB1 receptor occupation as a consequence of the sustained use of cannabis can trigger a process of desensitization, rendering subjects tolerant to the central and peripheral effects of Δ9-THC and other cannabinoid agonists (Gonzalez et al., 2005). Animals exposed repeatedly to Δ9-THC display decreased CB1 receptor levels as well as impaired coupling between CB1 and its transducing G-proteins (Gonzalez et al., 2005). Similarly, in humans, imaging studies have shown that chronic cannabis use leads to a down-regulation of CB1 receptors in the cortical regions of the brain and that this effect can be reversed by abstinence (Hirvonen et al., 2012).

CANNABINOID-BASED MEDICATIONS

The U.S. Food and Drug Administration (FDA) has licensed three drugs based on cannabinoids (see Table 2-2). Dronabinol, the generic name for synthetic Δ9-THC, is marketed under the trade name of Marinol® and is clinically indicated to counteract the nausea and vomiting associated with chemotherapy and to stimulate appetite in AIDS patients affected by wasting syndrome. A synthetic analog of Δ9-THC, nabilone (Cesamet®), is prescribed for similar indications. Both dronabinol and nabilone are given orally and have a slow onset of action. In July 2016 the FDA approved Syndros®, a liquid formulation of dronabinol, for the treatment of patients experiencing chemotherapy-induced nausea and vomiting who have not responded to conventional antiemetic therapies. The agent is also indicated for treating anorexia associated with weight loss in patients with AIDS. Two additional cannabinoid-based medications have been examined by the FDA. Nabiximols (Sativex®) is an ethanol cannabis extract composed of Δ9-THC and CBD in a one-to-one ratio. Nabiximols is administered as an oromucosal spray and is indicated in the symptomatic relief of multiple sclerosis and as an adjunctive analgesic treatment in cancer patients (Pertwee, 2012). As of September 2016, nabiximols has been launched in 15 countries, including Canada, Germany, Italy, Spain, the United Kingdom, and has been approved in a further 12, but not in the United States.5 In response to the urgent need expressed by parents of children with intractable epilepsy, in 2013 the FDA allowed investigational new drug studies of Epidiolex®, a concentrated CBD oil (>98 percent CBD), also developed by GW Pharmaceuticals, as an anti-seizure medication for Dravet and Lennox-Gastaut syndromes.

SYNTHETIC CANNABINOIDS AS RECREATIONAL DRUGS

In addition to nabilone, many other synthetic cannabinoids agonists have been described and widely tested on experimental animals to investigate the consequences of cannabinoid receptor activation6 (e.g., CP-55940, WIN-55212-2, JWH-018) (Iversen, 2000; Pertwee, 2012). The therapeutic application of these highly potent molecules is limited by their CB1-mediated psychotropic side effects, which presumably provide the rationale for the illicit use of some of them as an alternative to cannabis (Wells and Ott, 2011). Preclinical and clinical data in support of this claim remain very limited, however. Internet-marketed products such as Spice, K2, and Eclipse are a blend of various types of plant material (typically herbs and spices) that have been sprayed with one of these synthetic cannabinoids (as well as other non-cannabinoid psychoactive drugs). Since 2009 more than 140 different synthetic cannabinoids have been identified in herbal mixtures consumed as recreational drugs. The synthetic cannabinoids used in "herbal mixtures" are chemically heterogeneous, most of them being aminoalkylindole derivatives such as naphthoylindoles (e.g., JWH-018 and JWH-210), cyclopropylindoles (e.g., UR-144, XLR-11), or quinoline esters (e.g., PB-22). They seem to appeal especially to young cannabis and polydrug users because they are relatively inexpensive, easily available through the Internet, and difficult to identify with standard immunoassay drug screenings. In contrast to Δ9-THC, which is a partial agonist of the CB1 receptor, many of the synthetic cannabinoids bind to CB1 receptors with high affinity and efficacy, which may also be associated with higher potential of toxicity (Hermanns-Clausen et al., 2016). According to the National Institute on Drug Abuse (NIDA, 2012, p. 2), people using these various blends have been admitted to Poison Control Centers reporting "rapid heart rate, vomiting, agitation, confusion, and hallucinations." Synthetic cannabinoids can also raise blood pressure and cause a reduced blood supply to the heart (myocardial ischemia), and in a few cases they have been associated with heart attacks. Regular users may experience withdrawal and symptoms of dependence (Tait et al., 2016).

CANNABIS CONTAMINANTS AND ADULTERANTS

The large economic potential and illicit aspect of cannabis has given rise to numerous potentially hazardous natural contaminants or artificial adulterants being reported in crude cannabis and cannabis preparations. Most frequent natural contaminants consist of degradation products, microbial contamination (e.g., fungi, bacteria), and heavy metals. These contaminants are usually introduced during cultivation and storage (McLaren et al., 2008). Growth enhancers and pest control chemicals are the most common risks to both the producer and the consumer. Cannabis can also be contaminated for marketing purposes. This usually entails adding substances (e.g., tiny glass beads, lead) to increase the weight of the cannabis product (Busse et al., 2008; Randerson, 2007) or adding psychotropic substances (e.g., tobacco, calamus) and cholinergic compounds to either enhance the efficacy of low-quality cannabis or to alleviate its side effects (McPartland et al., 2008). Additionally, some extraction and inhalation methods used for certain dosing formulations (tinctures, butane hash oil, "dabs") can result in substantial pesticide and solvent contamination (Thomas and Pollard, 2016).

Who Should NOT use Cannabis?

• Cannabis may be a co-factor in schizophrenia later in life

• If a history of psychosis or schizophrenia, suggested to avoid all mind-altering substances such as cocaine, methamphetamines, cannabis

Addiction Issues?

• Addiction has not been found to be physical addiction, like heroin, nicotine and alcohol.

• May develop a psychological component of addiction. Use of the non-psychotropic topicals or sub-lingual can often be substituted

Cannabis is an herb with healing properties. These are exciting times to change our practices, promote change in clients/patients to more integrative medicine, and spread the word about a medicine that has few contraindications and fewer side effects than pharmaceuticals prescriptions. In my humble opinion, stay away from the real drugs.

• Not yet practical within the majority of hospitals or healthcare centers

• Use of edibles and topicals [creams, balms, sprays] has become more popular and in great demand because of their non-psychotropic effect.

Depending on the state, Nurse Practitioners are allow to assess patients and suggest Cannabis for specific disorders (ANA 2016). It is important to note that Cannabis is still illegal on the Federal level.

Side Effects?
• Munchies

• Sleep

• Temporary Paranoia

• Relaxation

• Dry mouth

• Decreased cognitive skills

- Rare side effects: unusual perception s of all senses, anxiety, hallucinations, slight increase in heart rate

- Study in LA of 1,252 smokers: a lung protective. Not associated with an increased risk of lung cancer

varies greatly among patients, even when treating the same condition.

Another famous product obtained from Cannabis is the cbd oil. Cannabidiol oil is used for health purposes, but it is controversial. There is some confusion about what it is and the effect it has on the human body. Cannabidiol (CBD) may have some health benefits, but there may also be some risks. It is also not legal in every state.

About Texas Cannabis Healing

Texas Cannabis Healing is a medical marijuana practice located in Cypress, Texas, that serves clientele from all of Texas. Highly trained medical providers take a compassionate, holistic approach to treatments for men and women of all ages in a welcoming, friendly atmosphere.

Texas Cannabis Healing helps patients who are ill, injured, or suffer from disease or ongoing pain find symptom relief in a natural way.

The highly experienced doctors use medical marijuana to treat an array of common medical conditions, such as cancer, chronic pain, seizures, multiple sclerosis, and post-traumatic stress disorder (PTSD), as well as autism, intractable epilepsy, and other chronic conditions.

Highly trained medical professionals personalize treatments using medical marijuana to restore quality of life in patients without addictive or harsh medications or invasive surgery.

The Power of Cannabis: The Healing Ability of Cannabinoids

As the social norms around cannabis slowly evolve in the United States, so do the legalities surrounding this formerly controversial plant. America is finally catching up with many other countries around the world, and recognizing the healing capabilities ofcannabis sativa. Although still federally illegal, each year more states introduce laws allowing for legal medical and recreational use of the plant. This not only allows people to finally access the medicine they desperately need, but also allows medical researchers the ability to pursue further cannabis studies when they previously had been restricted.

Although the research from American institutes had been severely restricted until relatively recently, it hasn't stopped other research centers around the world (in places like Israel, Brazil, Spain and Italy) from picking up the trail. Nowadays, far from being a fringe alternative medicine, medical marijuana and cannabis derivatives, including cannabidiol (CBD), have been proven to fight many diseases and illnesses. Not only has cannabis been found to be equally as powerful as more traditional pharmaceuticals, it has often been found to have even higher potential and with little to no serious side effects. Just as each new secret of the cannabis plant is uncovered, more avenues are opened for future study. At the moment, the medical potential seems endless.

Just how does a plant have such a powerful effect on human health? It all comes down to something called cannabinoids and the endocannabinoid system. One of the most important systems within our bodies is called the endocannabinoid system, which is responsible for a host of biological processes. Some examples of what the endocannabinoid system controls are appetite, mood stability, memory, pain perception, the nervous system, and the immune system. Cannabinoid receptors are located throughout the body, specifically crowded around the nervous system, the digestive tract and within the brain, although you can find them less concentrated in other areas.

Cannabis plants are named after the myriad of phytocannabinoids that they contain. Depending on strain, cannabis can contain upwards of 100 different cannabinoids including THC and CBD which are commonly known. Other lesser known cannabinoids are only now being pursued by the medical community. These cannabinoids can interact with the human endocannabinoid system. Some are able to directly influence the cannabinoid receptors, while others (like CBD) interact in a much more complex manner.

Each individual cannabinoid has a special relationship with the endocannabinoid system, for example some are more beneficial to sleep, while others are proving more useful for cancer treatment. More interesting still, each strain of cannabis has a complex mix of these cannabinoids that work together as a whole plant medicine for even more powerful results than previously understood through individual use.

Cannabis and Being Stoned

Importantly, not every cannabinoid found within cannabis triggers the stoned feeling. In fact, only the most (in)famous compound, THC, is responsible for all the psychoactive experiences many people associate with the plant. Therefore, if the specific strain is not bred for a high THC content, there is no way to have a mind altering experience. Having low THC strains is extremely beneficial for people seeking to use cannabis as a medicine, especially for children, seniors, and even pets.

There are many avenues being explored by international research centers, and there are many areas that already have significant research demonstrating the healing potential of cannabinoids. With just enough space to cover a few points only, we focus on the most highly publicized and proven areas of the medical potential of cannabinoids.

Anti-Cancer

Despite what you might think, cannabinoids are not simply a new drug claiming to cure cancer. They have been scientifically proven time and time again to be extremely effective at targeting specific types of cancer cells in laboratory study and animal trials. Currently, CBD specifically has been shown to slow cancer cell invasiveness, metastasis, cell division and cell migration. The evidence is so powerful, that many large pharmaceutical companies are trying to get ahead of the game and patent different cannabinoids for use as new cancer medications.

Anti-Seizure

Perhaps one of the areas with the most media coverage, strains high in CBD have been found to be extremely beneficial in treating drug-resistant forms of epilepsy. This has been especially true for children, as CBD doesn't cause any harmful side effects that can be common with other drugs. In some cases, CBD has been shown to dramatically reduce or even eliminate the appearance of seizures in children who had been having dozens of seizures a day.

Depression and Anxiety

The non-psychoactive cannabinoids found within cannabis often have counter effects to the psychoactivity of THC. For instance, CBD actually reduces appetite stimulation and anxiety: two common effects of THC heavy strains. On top of this, cannabinoids have been found to be equally, if not more, effective as treatment for depression and anxiety because they stimulate the SSRI receptors within the brain.

Anti-Inflammatory

For patients seeking relief from inflammatory diseases like irritable bowel syndrome and arthritis, cannabinoids may be able to provide an effective alternative. This is because they are an extremely powerful anti-inflammatory agent that targets the nervous system, and specifically the perception of pain.

Chronic Pain

Continuing on the above train of thought, cannabis is a welcome alternative for people seeking non-opioid forms of pain relief. Opioids come with a huge set of risks, including addiction, overdose, and severe constipation, but in recent studies, cannabinoids have been found to be equally as effective for long term pain relief without any of the issues associated with opioids.

WHAT IS CBD OIL?

CBD is one of many compounds, known as cannabinoids, that are found in the cannabis plant. Researchers have been looking at the potential therapeutic uses of CBD. Oils that contain concentrations of CBD are known as CBD oils. The concentration and uses of different oils vary.

Is CBD marijuana?

CBD oil is a cannabinoid derived from the cannabis plant.

Until recently, the most well-known compound in cannabis was delta-9 tetrahydrocannabinol (THC). This is the most active ingredient in marijuana.

Marijuana contains both THC and CBD, but the compounds have different effects.

THC is well-known for the mind-altering "high" it produces when broken down by heat and introduced into the body, such as when smoking the plant or cooking it into foods. Unlike THC, CBD is not psychoactive. This means that it does not change the state of mind of the person who uses it. However, it does appear to produce significant changes in the body and has been found to have medical benefits.

Most of the CBD used medicinally is found in the least processed form of the cannabis plant, known as hemp. Hemp and marijuana come from the same plant, cannabis sativa, but they are very different. Over the years, marijuana farmers have selectively bred their plants to be very high in THC and other compounds that interested them, either for a smell or an effect they had on the plant's flowers. On the other hand, hemp farmers have not tended to modify the plant. It is these hemp plants that are used to create CBD oil.

HOW CBD WORKS

All cannabinoids, including CBD, attach themselves to certain receptors in the body to produce their effects. The human body produces certain cannabinoids on its own. It has two receptors for cannabinoids, called CB1 receptors and CB2 receptors.

CB1 receptors are found all around the body, but many of them are in the brain. The CB1 receptors in the brain deal with coordination and movement, pain, emotions and mood, thinking, appetite, and memories, among others. THC attaches to these receptors.

CB2 receptors are more common in the immune system. They affect inflammation and pain. It used to be thought that CBD acts on these CB2 receptors, but it appears now that CBD does not act on either receptor directly. Instead, it seems to influence the body to use more of its own cannabinoids.

BENEFITS OF CBD

Because of the way that CBD acts in the body, it has many potential benefits. Natural pain relief or anti-inflammatory properties. People commonly use prescription or over-the-counter drugs to relieve pain and stiffness, including chronic pain.

Some people feel that CBD offers a more natural way to lower pain. A study published in the Journal of Experimental Medicine found that CBD significantly reduced chronic inflammation and pain in some mice and rats. The researchers suggest that the non-psychoactive compounds in marijuana, such as CBD, could be a new treatment for chronic pain.

Quitting smoking and drug withdrawals

There is some promising evidence that CBD use may help people to quit smoking. A pilot study posted to Addictive Behaviors found that smokers who used an inhaler containing the compound CBD smoked fewer cigarettes but did not have any additional craving for nicotine. Another similar study posted to Neurotherapeutics found that CBD may be a promising substance for people who abuse opioids.

Researchers noted that some symptoms experienced by patients with substance use disorders might be reduced by CBD. These include anxiety, mood symptoms, pain, and insomnia. These are early findings, but they suggest that CBD may be used to avoid or reduce withdrawal symptoms.

Epilepsy and other mental health disorders

CBD is also being studied for its possible role in treating epilepsy and neuropsychiatric disorders. A review posted to Epilepsia noted that CBD has anti-seizure properties and a low risk of side effects for people with epilepsy. Studies into CBD's effect on neurological disorders suggest that it may help to treat many of the disorders that are linked to epilepsy, such as neurodegeneration, neuronal injury, and psychiatric diseases. Another study published in Current Pharmaceutical Design found that CBD may have similar effects to certain antipsychotic drugs and that it may be safe and effective in treating patients with schizophrenia.

More research is needed to understand how this works, however.

Helps fight cancer

CBD has been studied for its use as an anti-cancer agent. A review posted to the British Journal of Clinical Pharmacology notes that CBD appears to block cancer cells from spreading around the body and invading an area entirely. The review indicates that this compound tends to suppress the growth of cancer cells and promote the death of these cells.

Researchers note that CBD may help in cancer treatment because of its low toxicity levels. They call for it to be studied along with standard treatments, to check for synergistic effects.

Anxiety disorders

Patients with chronic anxiety are often advised to avoid cannabis, as THC can trigger or amplify anxiety and paranoia in some people. However, a review from Neurotherapeutics suggests that CBD may help to reduce the anxiety felt by people with certain anxiety disorders.

The researchers point to studies showing that CBD may reduce anxiety behaviors in disorders such as:

- post-traumatic stress disorder
- general anxiety disorder
- panic disorder
- social anxiety disorder
- obsessive-compulsive disorder

The review notes that current medications for these disorders can lead to additional symptoms and side effects and that people may stop taking the drugs because of these unwanted effects. CBD has not shown any adverse effects in these cases to date, and the researchers call for CBD to be studied as a potential treatment method.

Type 1 diabetes

Type 1 diabetes is caused by inflammation when the immune system attacks cells in the pancreas. Recent research posted to Clinical Hemorheology and Microcirculation found that CBD may ease the inflammation in the pancreas in type 1 diabetes. This may be the first step in finding a CBD-based treatment for type 1 diabetes.

Acne

Acne treatment is another promising use for CBD. The condition is caused, in part, by inflammation and overworked sebaceous glands in the body. A recent study posted to the Journal of Clinical Investigation found that CBD helps to lower the production of sebum that leads to acne, partly because of its anti-inflammatory effect on the body. CBD could be a future treatment for acne vulgaris, the most common form of acne.

Alzheimer's disease

Initial research published in the Journal of Alzheimer's Disease found that CBD was able to prevent the development of social recognition deficit in subjects. This means that CBD could potentially prevent people in the early stages of Alzheimer's from losing their ability to recognize the faces of people that they know. This is the first evidence that CBD has potential to prevent Alzheimer's disease symptoms.

AILMENTS CURED

AIDS/HIV

In a human study of 10 HIV-positive marijuana smokers, scientists found people who smoked marijuana ate better, slept better and experienced a better mood. Another small study of 50 people found patients that smoked cannabis saw less neuropathic pain.

Alzheimer's

Medical marijuana and some of the plant's chemicals have been used to help Alzheimer's patients gain weight, and research found that it lessens some of the agitated behavior that patients can exhibit. In one cell study, researchers found it slowed the progress of protein deposits in the brain. Scientists think these proteins may be part of what causes Alzheimer's, although no one knows what causes the disease.

Arthritis

A study of 58 patients using the derivatives of marijuana found they had less arthritis pain and slept better. Another review of studies concluded marijuana may help fight pain-causing inflammation.

Asthma

Studies are contradictory, but some early work suggests it reduced exercise-induced asthma. Other cell studies showed smoking marijuana could dilate human airways, but some patients experienced a tight feeling in their chests and throats. A study in mice found similar results.

Cancer

Animal studies have shown some marijuana extracts may kill certain cancer cells. Other cell studies show it may stop cancer growth, and with mice, THC, the psychoactive ingredient in marijuana, improved the impact of radiation on cancer cells. Marijuana can also prevent the nausea that often accompanies chemotherapy treatment used to treat cancer.

Chronic pain

Some animal and small human studies show that cannabinoids can have a "substantial analgesic effect." People widely used them for pain relief in the 1800s. Some medicines based on cannabis such as Sativex are being tested on multiple sclerosis patients and used to treat cancer pain. The drug has been approved in Canada and in some European countries. In another trial involving 56 human patients, scientists saw a 30% reduction in pain in those who smoked marijuana.

Crohn's disease

In a small pilot study of 13 patients watched over three months, researchers found inhaled cannabis did improve life for people suffering from ulcerative colitis and Crohn's disease. It helped ease people's pain, limited the frequency of diarrhea and helped with weight gain.

Epilepsy

Medical marijuana extract in early trials at the NYU Langone Medical Center showed a 50% reduction in the frequency of certain seizures in children and adults in a study of 213 patients recently.

Glaucoma

Glaucoma is one of the leading causes of blindness. Scientists have looked at THC's impact on this disease on the optic nerve and found it can lower eye pressure, but it may also lower blood pressure, which could harm the optic nerve due to a reduced blood supply. THC can also help preserve the nerves, a small study found.

Multiple sclerosis

Using marijuana or some of the chemicals in the plant may help prevent muscle spasms, pain, tremors and stiffness, according to early-stage, mostly observational studies involving animals, lab tests and a small number of human patients. The downside — it may impair memory, according to a small study involving 20 patients.

Method

Medicinal marijuana is either smoked or the extracts are taken orally.

The basic principal for dosing medical marijuana is to start with a low dose and to go slow in taking more until the effect of the first dose is fully realized, because the effects of cannabis are not always immediately felt. Starting low and going slow allows patients to accommodate for the different experiences they may have. Cannabis has a wide margin of safety and there is limited risk of overdose. However, caution is warranted until a patient fully understands the effect that the cannabis may have. Dosag

Cannabis is legal for either medicinal or recreational use in some but not all states. Other states approve CBD oil as a hemp product without approving the general use of medical marijuana. Laws may differ between federal and state level, and current marijuana and CBD legislation in the United States can be confusing, even in states where marijuana is legal.

There is an ever-changing number of states that do not necessarily consider marijuana to be legal but have laws directly related to CBD oil. This information is up to date as of July 24, 2017, but the laws frequently change.

The laws vary, but they generally approve CBD oil as legal for treating a range of epileptic conditions at various concentrations. A full list of states that have CBD-specific laws is available here.

Different states also require different levels of prescription to possess and use CBD oil. In Missouri, for example, a person must show that three other treatment options have been unsuccessful in treating epilepsy. If you are considering CBD oil as a treatment for a suitable condition, talk to your local healthcare provider. They will have an understanding of safe CBD sources and local laws surrounding usage. Research the laws for your own state. In most cases, a prescription will be required.

Side effects

Many small-scale studies have looked into the safety of CBD in adults and found that it is well tolerated across a wide range of doses. There have been no significant side effects in the central nervous system or effects on vital signs and mood among people who use it either slightly or heavily. The most common side effect noted is tiredness. Some people have noticed diarrhea and changes in appetite or weight.

Risks

There are still very little long-term safety data available, and, to date, tests have not been carried out on children. As with any new or alternative treatment option, a patient should discuss CBD with a qualified healthcare practitioner before use.

The United States Food and Drug Administration (FDA) has not approved CBD for the treatment of any condition. It can be difficult to know whether a product contains a safe or effective level of CBD or whether the product has the properties and contents stated on its packaging and marketing.

HOW TO USE

CBD oil is used in different ways to relieve the symptoms of different conditions. Some CBD oil products can be mixed into different foods or drinks, taken from a pipette or dropper, or are available as a thick paste to be massaged into the skin. CBD can also be purchased in capsule form. Other products are provided as sprays that are meant to be administered under the tongue. Here are a few recommended dosages, although these may vary between individuals based on other factors, such as body weight, the concentration of the product, and the condition being treated. Due to the lack of FDA regulation for CBD products, seek advice from a medical professional before settling on any particular dosage.

All dosages relate to taking CBD oil by mouth. These can include:

- Chronic pain: Take between 2.5 and 20 milligrams (mg) by mouth for no more than 25 days.

- Epilepsy: Consume between 200 and 300 mg of CBD by mouth daily for up to 4.5 months.

- Movement problems associated with Huntington's disease: Taking 10 mg every day for six weeks can help ease movements.

- Sleep disorders: Take between 40 and 160 mg.

- Schizophrenia: Consume between 40 and 1,280 mg CBD by mouth daily for up to 4 weeks.

- Glaucoma: One dose of between 20 and 40 mg applied under the tongue can help to relieve pressure in the eye. However, caution is advised – doses greater than 40 mg might actually increase pressure.

As regulation in the U.S. increases, more exact doses and prescriptions will start to emerge.

After discussing dosage and risks with a doctor, and researching regional legal use, it is important to compare different brands. There are a range of different CBD oils available to purchase online, with different benefits and applications.

15 reasons edible cannabis heals

1) Cancer Prevention

The edible forms of the marijuana plant have been used for thousands of years. One of their most unique health benefits is their potential capacity to oxidize free radicals in the body, suggesting that they may help prevent cancer. Cannabidiol (CBD) reduces tumor growth and stimulates apoptosis in animal models as well as inhibiting cell proliferation and invasion.

2) Alleviates Anxiety

Marijuana edibles can assist with several anxiety problems, and THC and CBD might help you get a better night's sleep. It is known that marijuana edibles aid in the promotion of healthy sleep for individuals who struggle with bouts of Social Anxiety Disorder. Edibles' soothing effects will help you relax in most situations and cut down on your stress levels when every day feels like an uphill battle.

3) Pain Relief

The cannabinoids present in cannabis have been shown to be effective for pain relief. A single dose of THC reduced neuropathic pain in cancer patients within minutes. CBD has also demonstrated anti-inflammatory and analgesic effects in multiple human studies. It is currently being used to treat chronic pain.

4) Migraine Relief

Marijuana edibles are also used to relieve pain, notably migraines. Edible marijuana products can treat various types of chronic pain and have been shown to be especially effective in reducing neuropathic pain. This is because the cannabinoids in marijuana bind to cannabinoid receptors in the central nervous system. Cannabinoid receptors are involved in the sensation of pain, which makes marijuana edibles an effective treatment for migraines.

5) Treats Nausea

THC has anti-nausea effects on chemotherapy patients and is also about as effective as prochlorperazine (Compazine) at combating nausea and vomiting after surgery or other medical procedures. When combined with antipsychotic medication, marijuana has been proven to reduce the debilitating effects of nausea and vomiting in cancer and AIDS patients.

6) Epilepsy Relief

For epilepsy patients, CBD can help control seizures and stop them from spreading which is why many sufferers may benefit from ingesting marijuana edibles rather than smoking the leaves. A 2003 case study reported successful treatment with marijuana on subjects who were not responsive to traditional medical treatment. Smoking cannabis reduced seizure frequency in more than 50 percent of patients and stopped seizures altogether in nine subjects.

7) Stops Cancer Cells From Spreading

One way that cancer spreads is through cell migration, which can result in metastasis or tumors invading other tissues and organs around the body. CBD has been shown to suppress cell migration in cancer cells, meaning that it could help stop the spread of cancer.

8) Addiction Recovery

In the rehabilitation sector, marijuana use is still understandably contentious, however medicinal marijuana's legality has opened the door to a new method of withdrawal from harmful medications such as opioids and narcotics.

Cannabis is sometimes suggested as a method to get off of addictive drugs like heroin and lessen the impact of quitting. Edibles are a more appealing alternative to opioids or other deadly, habit-forming chemicals, and they are typically healthier than methadone or buprenorphine therapy. When attempting to leave any addiction, please contact your doctor or recovery specialist for a personalized plan.

9) Digestive Aid

Marijuana edibles are also effective for treating digestive problems. The cannabinoids present in cannabis stimulate gastric juices and intestinal muscles, which help with digestion and prevent conditions like constipation. They can also help with the absorption of food and nutrients, which is especially beneficial for those suffering from conditions like Crohn's Disease or Irritable Bowel Syndrome.

10) Stimulates Appetite

Marijuana edibles are often used to stimulate appetite in patients who have lost their hunger due to medical treatments like chemotherapy or radiation therapy. However, it can also be used to curb anorexia in patients suffering from HIV/AIDS or other diseases.

11) Weight Loss

Marijuana has been shown to help people lose weight in a healthy way. Cannabis sativa strains have been shown to increase metabolism and stimulate the appetite in a way that promotes weight loss. The cannabinoids found in cannabis activate the cannabinoid receptors, which leads to a reduction in food intake.

12) Vegetarian Alternative to Fish Oils

Cannabis is a healthy alternative source of omega-3 fatty acids, which are extremely beneficial when consumed.

They reduce inflammation and help fight off cancer and neurodegenerative diseases like Alzheimer's. Without the risk of mercury contamination in fish oils, it's a much healthier choice for many people.

13) Protects Bone Density

According to a 2014 study, CBD can help protect against bone deterioration that results from osteoporosis. Some researchers believe that the anti-inflammatory properties of marijuana could even be helpful in treating arthritis. However, this would need to be confirmed on an individual basis with your doctor first.

14) Anti Inflammatory

Most of the benefits of edible cannabis are due to its anti-inflammatory properties. By fighting off inflammation, these benefits can help protect against conditions like osteoporosis and liver disease.

15) Protection Against Alzheimer's Disease

CBD has been shown to have protective effects on the nervous system, which could be beneficial in slowing down or preventing the onset of Alzheimer's Disease. CBD has also been shown to reduce anxiety and depression in

Alzheimer's patients, which are common co-morbidities of the disease.

CHAPTER TWO

Basic Healing Cannabis Salve

This is a recipe for a Basic Cannabis Salve you can make at home. Easy to customize to your own needs.

Equipment

- Double-boiler or pot with a glass bowl that can sit firmly on top
- Grinder or food processor (optional)
- Cheesecloth
- Metal colander or ricer
- Glass bowl
- Rubber or silicone spatula
- Kitchen towel
- Storage containers with lids

Materials

- 1/2 oz Dried cannabis flowers, leaves and stems
- 1 1/2 cups Organic virgin coconut oil Or the oil of your choice
- 1/2 cup Avocado oil Or the oil of your choice

- 3-5 Tbsp. Beeswax pastilles (or 1.5-2.5 oz grated) See post for why this varies

- 2 Tbsp. Liquid or granulated lecithin

- 1/4 oz Dried companion herbs of your choice (by weight)

- 1 Tbsp Essential oils of your choice No more than 1 Tbsp. total of essential oils

- 1 Tbsp Infused oils of your choice No more than 1 Tbsp. of infused oils

- Cannabis Infusion

- Bring several inches of water to a boil in the pan portion of the double-boiler.

ALTERNATIVE 1: Use a glass bowl that fits snugly over a pot of boiling water instead.

ALTERNATIVE 2: Use a crock pot on the "Keep Warm" setting without water.

Once the water is boiling, reduce heat to low.

Add the coconut oil to the pot and allow it to melt.

Add avocado oil and cannabis.

OPTIONAL: Add any dried companion herbs at this time.

Continue to cook over low-heat, stirring every once in awhile, for approximately 3-4 hours. The oil should turn a dark-green and your house should be fragrant!

IMPORTANT Double-boilers WILL lose water overtime. Be sure to check it every hour and add BOILING water if necessary to the water level up.

Remove from heat. Allow oils and cannabis to cool for 15-20 minutes.

Fold the cheesecloth into thirds, allowing enough material to drape over the sides of your colander. Place the colander over your glassbowl.

Slowly pour the infused oils into the cheesecloth covered colander. Use a spoon to push gently on the flowers to extract more oil.

Carefully gather the corners of the cheesecloth up before squeezing as much oil out as possible. The remaining oil should have very little if any solid matter left in in.

ALTERNATIVE: Use the cheesecloth in the ricer instead to expel oil from the plant matter.

Ensure the bowl of the double-boiler is free of any solid matter. Wipe it out with a paper towel if needed, then wipe that on any achy parts of your body! I don't like to waste any of it 🙂

Popularity

Weed is popular worldwide, but not for its medicinal uses. Its medicinal benefits are reaped by only a few but thanks to many protests marijuana is now legal in countries like Canada and England. On the other hand, countries like India continue to treat it at illegal.

Controversies

Cannabis, or marijuana, is famous as a recreational drug, used commonly to 'get high' hence its legalization has become a topic of great controversy. Some countries have legalized it, like Canada, because of its medicinal uses, while others have refused to do so.

Salve Making

Bring the water in the double-boiler (or pot with glass bowl firmly set on top) back up to a boil before reducing the heat to low.

Pour your infused oil back in to the top part of the double-boiler or in the glass bowl.

Add beeswax and lecithin, stirring to incorporate them as they melt.

Continue stirring for 5 minutes after everything has melted.

Use a spoon to gather up a sample of the salve. Place the spoon on a plate in the freezer for 2-3 minutes. Bring it out and check the consistency- it should require a little pressure to get through it. If it's still runny, add more beeswax 1/2 ounce at a time until you reach a desired consistency.

Turn off the stove and place a folded up kitchen towel on the counter. Remove the bowl of the double-boiler carefully and place it on the towel to avoid any moisture burning you or getting in the salve. Add Vitamin-E oil and gently stir to incorporate. If you are adding any other essential oils, now is the time.

As you stir, close your eyes and focus your energy and intentions on the salve. I like to focus on imagery that conveys healing. You may laugh, but I find this step important!

Pour the finished salve in to clean containers and place the lid on. This will make approximately 18-20 ounces, depending on how much oil the dried cannabis soaked up and how much beeswax used.

Call everyone in your family over to where you are working. Use the spatula to scrape up every last bit of salve and rub it all over your bodies.

The Effects of Cannabis on Your Body

Respiratory system

Much like tobacco smoke, cannabis smoke is made up of a variety of toxic chemicals, including ammonia and hydrogen cyanide, which can irritate your bronchial passages and lungs.

If you're a regular smoker, you're more likely to wheeze, cough, and produce phlegm. You're also at an increased risk of bronchitis and lung infections. Cannabis may aggravate existing respiratory illnesses, such as asthma and cystic fibrosis.

Cannabis and COPD: Is there a link?

Cannabis smoke contains carcinogens, which could theoretically increase your risk of lung cancer.

However, according to the National Institute of Drug Abuse (NIDA), there is no conclusive evidence that cannabis smoke causes lung cancer. More research is needed.

THC moves from your lungs into your bloodstream and throughout your body. Within minutes, your heart rate may increase by 20 to 50 beats per minute. That rapid heart rate can continue for up to 3 hours.

This places extra oxygen demand on your heart. If you have heart disease, this could raise your risk for a heart attack.

One of the telltale signs of recent cannabis use is bloodshot eyes. The eyes look red because cannabis causes blood vessels to expand and fill with more blood.

THC can also lower pressure in the eyes, which can ease symptoms of glaucoma for a few hours. More research is needed to understand whether THC can offer long-term benefits for glaucoma.

Central nervous system

The effects of cannabis extend throughout the central nervous system (CNS). Cannabis is thought to ease pain and inflammation and help control spasms and seizures.

Still, there are potential long-term negative effects on the CNS to consider.

THC triggers your brain to release large amounts of dopamine, a naturally occurring "feel good" chemical. It's what gives you a pleasant high. It may heighten your sensory perception and your perception of time.

This dopamine cycle may also explain why as many as 30 percent of cannabis users develop cannabis use disorder. Severe cannabis use disorder, or addiction, may be relatively uncommon, but it can occur.

Symptoms of cannabis withdrawal may include:
- irritability
- insomnia
- loss of appetite

In the hippocampus, THC changes the way you process information, so your judgment may be impaired. The hippocampus is responsible for memory, so it may also be difficult to form new memories when you're high.

Changes also take place in the cerebellum and basal ganglia. These brain areas play roles in movement and balance. Cannabis may alter your balance, coordination, and reflex response. All those changes mean that it's not safe to drive.

Very large doses of cannabis or high concentrations of THC can cause hallucinations or delusions. According to the NIDA, there may be an association between cannabis use and some mental health conditions like depression and anxiety.

You may want to avoid cannabis if you have schizophrenia or a family history of schizophrenia. Cannabis may make symptoms worse or increase the chances of developing the condition in people who have a genetic predisposition.

When you come down from the high, you may feel tired or a bit depressed. In some people, cannabis can cause anxiety.

In people younger than 25 years, whose brains haven't yet fully developed, long-term cannabis use can have a lasting detrimental impact on thinking and memory processes.

Using cannabis during pregnancy can also affect the developing baby. The child may have trouble with memory, concentration, and problem-solving skills.

As mentioned earlier, federal prohibition has made research into the effects of cannabis largely observational, which can only detect correlation and not causation.

Moreover, these studies were generally looking at unregulated, illegal cannabis, and scientists don't know whether legal cannabis regulated by states has different effects.

Digestive system

Smoking cannabis can cause some stinging or burning in your mouth and throat while you're inhaling.

Cannabis can cause digestive issues when taken orally. While THC has been shown to ease nausea and vomiting, in some people long-term heavy use can paradoxically cause nausea and vomiting.

An increase in your appetite is common when taking any form of THC, leading to what many people call "the munchies."

This can be a benefit for people who need to gain weight or increase appetite, such as people with cancer receiving chemotherapy.

For others who are looking to lose weight, this effect could be considered a disadvantage, although epidemiological studies suggest cannabis users don't have increased risk for diabetes or obesity compared with nonusers.

Immune system

Studies involving animals have shown that THC may adversely affect the immune system by suppressing it.

This could theoretically make you more susceptible to infectious diseases. However, for people with autoimmune conditions who have an overactive immune system, this may be a benefit.

Health Risks of Cannabis Use

Knowledge about cannabis and its impacts is constantly evolving. The majority of people who use cannabis do not suffer any negative consequences. However, various factors seem to contribute to negative effects in some people.

Risk factors

- Risks to cognitive abilities

- Physical health risks

- Mental health risks

- Risks of regular use

- Risks of mixing cannabis with other substances

- Risks during pregnancy and while breastfeeding

Risk factors

Although problems may occur for first-time cannabis users, issues related to physical and mental health mainly arise as a result of repeated use over several months or years. Accidents and injuries, on the other hand, may occur as a result of one-time or occasional use. Certain factors can increase or reduce a cannabis user's risk of being negatively affected:

- A personal or family history of mental health issues such as psychosis and bipolar disorder

- Frequency of use: Regular use (once a week or more) is often linked to increased risk of health problems

- Type of product used: Products with higher THC content may be more harmful

- The age at which a person starts to use cannabis: use during adolescence is generally associated with an increased risk of negative effects

The circumstances of use, for example:

- When cannabis is combined with other substances such as alcohol or medications

- When an individual has personal responsibilities such as work or the supervision of children

The method of use: Smoking cannabis appears to be more risky than other methods of use, although poisoning from foods containing cannabis is common among inexperienced users.

However, caution should be exercised before attributing the cause of a health problem to cannabis use. It is possible that the problem:

- Was already present prior to cannabis use

- Is a result of cannabis use

- Is influenced by cannabis use or, conversely, influences cannabis use

Based on these factors, it is difficult to predict whether or not an individual will experience significant problems after using cannabis. Most experts agree that cannabis use is never 100% safe.

Risks to cognitive abilities

The health risks and negative health impacts of cannabis use stem from its effects on cognitive abilities, such as:

- Judgement

- Attention span

- Memory

- The ability to make decisions

These effects can impact daily activities such as:
- Driving a car

- Work

- Learning activities

Other situations that require coordination and speed

Cannabis begins to take effect within minutes of being inhaled, and a little later if ingested. The effects often last for several hours and are usually reversible. Some studies suggest that reduced cognitive function may persist longer in the event of sustained and repeated use, especially if it begins in adolescence.

Cannabis use can exacerbate some existing health problems, such as chronic diseases:

- Cannabis use increases the heart rate and can alter its rhythm. It also increases blood pressure.
- Inhaling cannabis smoke can aggravate existing respiratory diseases and even promote disease onset.
- Like tobacco smoke, cannabis smoke contains a number of substances that are harmful to your health, including some carcinogens.
- However, the most recent scientific studies do not prove that the risk of developing lung, throat, or neck cancer is higher among cannabis users.

Also, cannabis vaping is associated with a risk of developing an acute lung disease. This practice should be avoided. To learn more about the risks associated with vaping cannabis, see the warning against vaping cannabis This link will open in a new window. (in French only) on the website of the Ministère de la Santé et des Services sociaux.

Mental health risks

Psychotic symptoms

Individuals who are under the influence of cannabis may experience psychotic symptoms such as:

- Hallucinations with false visual, auditory, and/or tactile perceptions

- Paranoid ideas that seem detached from reality

- In most cases, these psychotic experiences are limited to when the person is intoxicated and disappear on their own. Other individuals may experience persistent, long-term, and much more serious symptoms. According to experts, cannabis use does not cause psychotic disorders, but it can be a contributing factor for some people.

Individuals who regularly use cannabis may show a lack of interest in activities other than using cannabis (studies, work, leisure, etc.). They may also experience symptoms of depression This link will open in a new window., for example:

- Deep sadness
- Fatigue
- Irritability
- Sense of worthlessness

Some individuals with depression may be tempted to use cannabis to relieve their symptoms. To date, scientific evidence has not shown that cannabis is effective in treating depression. Using it for this purpose is not recommended.

Some studies suggest that cannabis users experience symptoms of anxiety more frequently than non-users However, it is difficult to predict whether or not cannabis will influence their anxiety levels. Some people may experience panic attacks when they use cannabis, while others find it relaxing.

Problematic cannabis use

Cannabis use can be problematic if people lose control of their use and suffer negative consequences in various spheres of their life as a result. Some people may become addicted to cannabis, as it is the case with other substances. Individuals may:

- Develop a tolerance to the substance (i.e., need to use more to feel the same effect)
- Experience withdrawal symptoms when they reduce or stop use
- Have a strong desire to use
- Be unable to stop using
- Spend a significant portion of their time buying or using cannabis or recovering from cannabis use
- Use repeatedly in such a way that it prevents them from fulfilling important obligations at work, school, or home

- Use despite personal and/or social problems related to use

- Reduce or give up social, professional, or leisure activities as a result of use

About 1 in 11 people who use cannabis will develop a problematic use of cannabis in their lifetime. Among adolescents, 1 in 6 users will develop addiction problematic use. Use of and addiction to other products including alcohol and tobacco are more common among cannabis users.

Research has also established the existence of a cannabis withdrawal syndrome. It occurs when regular cannabis users significantly reduce or stop cannabis use. Symptoms include:

- Restlessness

- Irritability

- Sleep problems, which may last a number of weeks after stopping use

Risks of regular use

The health risks of cannabis use increase with both the frequency (e.g., number of times used in a week) and duration of use (e.g., number of years used).

Risks of mixing cannabis with other substances

Cannabis and Alcohol

Whenever you drink alcohol or take a drug, the effect This link will open in a new window. the substance will have on you is always a bit unknown. Mixing alcohol with recreational or prescription drugs increases the likelihood of harmful effects. That's why a lot of cannabis users drink little or no alcohol when they consume cannabis. They know the two don't mix.

Mixing cannabis with alcohol further reduces your ability to drive a vehicle.

Cannabis and Tobacco

Mixing cannabis and tobacco isn't a good idea either. Their combined use presents a greater health risk—not to mention that tobacco is highly addictive.

Cannabis can have an impact on the effect of the medication you're taking. The inverse is also true: some medications can alter the effects of cannabis. Before consuming cannabis, ask a health professional if there are any known interactions with your medications.

Risks during pregnancy and while breastfeeding

When a mother consumes cannabis, the THC winds up in the placenta she's carrying and in her breast milk. Since the short- and long-term effects of THC exposure on fetuses and babies are currently unknown, it's best to avoid cannabis and cannabis-derived products and exposure to secondhand smoke if you're pregnant or breastfeeding. If you're having a hard time giving up cannabis, talk to a trusted health professional.

7 Potential Health Benefits of Cannabis

1. Lowering blood pressure

A study conducted by JCI Insight in 2017 found that CBD lowered the blood pressure of human participants. It reduced their resting blood pressure as well as their blood pressure after stress tests including mental arithmetic, isometric exercise, and the cold pressor test.

2. Reducing inflammation

CBD has been proven to help reduce inflammation and the neuropathic pain it can cause, according to a study by the Rockefeller Institute of Medical Research.

3. Preventing relapse in drug and alcohol addiction

A 2018 study discovered that CBD can be useful in helping people who suffer from drug and alcohol addiction. A preclinical trial with lab rats determined that CBD reduced the stress-induced cravings, anxiety and lack of impulse control that often cause people to relapse.

4. Treating anxiety disorders

Anxiety is perhaps the most common affliction that people have used CBD for, and a preclinical study found that CBD could be effective in treating generalized anxiety disorder, panic disorder, social anxiety disorder, obsessive-compulsive disorder, and post-traumatic stress disorder.

5. Treating gastrointestinal (GI) disorders

A recent study found that CBD and other non-psychoactive cannabinoids can effectively be used to prevent and treat GI disorders such as irritable bowel syndrome (IBS), inflammatory bowel disease (IBD), Crohn's, ulcerative colitis and more. CBD's anti-inflammatory properties are key to reducing and preventing symptoms.

6. Preventing seizures

Decades of research have gone into using CBD to treat epilepsy and other seizure syndromes, and a recent study showed it can have positive effects in reducing symptoms and seizure frequency.

7. Fighting cancer

Not only has CBD been used to help alleviate the effects of chemotherapy, but studies have also found it can prevent cell growth and induce cell death in cervical cancer cell lines and it has numerous anti-cancer effects that can help prevent a variety of cancers, treat tumors, and benefit the immune system.

Beyond these seven benefits, there are even more still being researched and tested.

Pros and Cons of Cannabis Consumption

Pros

Helps Battling Addictions

Using eight major cannabinoids (substances within the cannabis strains), researchers treated people with the proclivity towards prescription drugs, cigarettes, alcohol, and heavy opioid addictions. The experiment resulted in up to 66% success rate, especially with prescription drug addiction.

This is not surprising because most cannabinoids do a great deal in treating anxiety, symptoms of Multiple Sclerosis, back pain, cancer pain, chemo side-effects, etc.

The United States National Institute of Health ran a study with 91 participants who were heavy opioid users, treating them with cannabis. Eventually, a large majority of them switched to cannabis.

It Blasts the Production of Osteoblasts

Essentially, osteoblasts are bone-producing cells which do the most work when it comes to healing broken or damaged bones. The CBD (cannabidiol) treatment does a great deal in helping the production of these cells, helping the bone re-grow roughly 40% faster and leaving it about 50% stronger than before.

Multiple sclerosis is a somewhat frequent disease in today's society, with some 2.3 million patients in the US only. A large number of them treat the side effects of this illness with CBD oils containing only 0.3% THC (tetrahydrocannabinol). It is a substance used for pain and anxiety relief.

Major cannabinoids help saving Beta cells (insulin-producing cells), battling even the highest Diabetes type 1 risks. Within the cannabis-consuming community, Diabetes type 2 is close to non-existent.

Getting diagnosed with a mental disorder oftentimes is followed by harsh prescription drug treatment, with major negative side effects on our body. For instance, HN (hippocampus neurogenesis) is a process of stimulation of both neuron creation and revitalization. This process is proven to be stimulated by the use of cannabinoids.

Also, approximately 90% of patients fighting depression and ADHD who were treated with CBD showed reduced symptoms of these issues, such as anxiety, insomnia, hyperactivity, loss of appetite, etc.

Helps With Overall Cancer Treatment

Even though the controversies surrounding this topic never cease, one thing is evident. The cannabinoid compounds, especially infused within CBD oil, tend to equip one's body for harsh chemo side-effects, like pain, vomiting, weight loss, body weakness, etc.

Cons

Using Cannabis Could Lead to Misuse And Addiction

Roughly 30% of people consuming cannabis have a type of use disorder, with often withdrawals such as shakiness, insomnia, depression, sweating, and visceral pain.

It Could Boost Cognitive Decline

This is a long-term and continuous side-effect, bringing eventual issues with learning and motoric skills in adults.

It Could Cause Lung And Oral Hygiene Issues

Even though there are clean ways of consuming cannabis, the vast amount of consumers smokes it. As a form of consumption, smoking causes cavities, mouth cancer, gingivitis, and neck cancer.

The toxic compounds inhaled through smoking, such as ammonia, hydrogen-cyanide, benzopyrene, and many others cause bronchial irritation, lung bleeding, and cancer.

It Has Bad Effects on Cardiovascular System

People with a history of heart issues are not encouraged toward cannabis use, as it can dilate their blood vessels, causing a possible cardiac arrest.

Its Use Was Connected With Paranoid Behavior And Schizophrenia Triggering

Oxford University published research which shows that 50% of those who took cannabis reported paranoid thoughts, as opposed to the 30% who were given a placebo substitute.

CONCLUSION

Cannabis is a powerful plant with many healing properties that have been ignored for far too long. When used correctly, edibles can provide relief from a variety of conditions and improve the quality of life for those suffering from them.

By now most people that have done any research on cannabis know that it is as healing as it is inspiring to the body. Many people enjoy rolling up a blunt or packing a bowl, but far too many individuals miss out on the exceptional healing and euphoric experience that comes with eating their favorite Kush cannabis in an infused edible.

The advantages of consuming this benevolent plant are numerous, whether medicinal or recreational type. It helps fighting anxiety, depression, chronic pain, insomnia, etc. However, it is important to thoroughly inform yourself before deciding to start consuming cannabis, as there are negative side effects as well.